Paleo Diet for Beginners

The Essential Guide to Getting Started with Paleo Diet

Contents

Introduction

The rising number of people diagnosed with celiac disease and gluten sensitivity has attracted more attention to the theory that our bodies are not genetically designed to eat grains. This theory is what has led to the popularity of the Paleolithic, Paleo or Stone Age diets.

There are some scientific studies that support this theory. It's true that until about 10,000 years ago, grains were not cultivated and so were not a part of the daily human diet. It's also true that people in pre-agricultural times did not seem to have suffered from various metabolic and digestive disorders that have been attributed to eating grains and processed foods such as breads, cereals, pastries and other modern favorites. The rate of metabolic syndrome, type 2 diabetes, obesity and other such disorders has risen dramatically in the past few decades, and many nutritionists and researchers blame the fact that processed grains make up a growing proportion of the typical daily diet.

Researchers and nutritionists who have recommended removing grains and legumes from our diets suggest that our bodies have not had enough time to adapt genetically to absorbing and processing grains. Since gluten comes from grains, it may follow that we're not genetically adapted to eating it, either.

The jury is still out on whether eating grains is bad for our health. But quite a few people have chosen to follow diets like the Paleo diet, which is a gluten-free diet that is also very high in protein. Many people following the Paleo diet report better digestive health, more energy and less inflammation.

Scientists can't confidently say that all grains are bad for your health. They do know that wheat, barley, rye and possibly oats are dangerous for those with celiac disease and gluten sensitivity, and that wheat and wheat products are a health threat to those with a wheat allergy.

Obviously, a Paleo diet is essential for those who have been diagnosed with either celiac disease or gluten sensitivity. It's also a simple option for those who have a wheat allergy, as it takes much of the guesswork and label-reading out of the equation. But is going gluten-free beneficial to the rest of us? The answer is maybe.

Disclaimer

No part of this eBook can be transmitted or reproduced in any form including print, electronic, photocopying, scanning, mechanical or recording without prior written permission from the author.

All information, ideas and guidelines presented here are for educational purposes only. While the author has taken utmost efforts to ensure the accuracy of the written content, all readers are advised to follow information mentioned herein at their own risk. The author cannot be held responsible for any personal or commercial damage caused by misinterpretation of information. All readers are encouraged to seek professional advice when needed.

1. Foundation

Eliminating or greatly reducing prepared or convenience foods from your diet is always a good thing. Many of these foods are high in fats, sugar and other ingredients that you simply don't need in a healthy diet — in any form. Empty calories (calories with little nutrition) come from heavily processed foods and snacks such as cookies, cakes, crackers, pasta, sugary cereals, buns and rolls. By not eating them, we can make our diets significantly healthier and more nutritious.

Eliminating Grains May Very Well Be a Good Idea

Researchers and scientists agree that humans have only been eating grains for less than 1 percent of our history as a species. There's still a good deal of debate about whether that fact has any significance when it comes to health and nutrition, but many well-respected nutritionists believe it does. Many followers of diets such as the Paleo diet agree, and they report feeling much better overall, with fewer digestive issues and headaches, and an increase in energy.

Weight Loss

A Paleo diet is not necessarily a weight-loss diet. In fact, if you're not careful, you could actually gain weight once you go gluten-free. It is possible to lose weight while on a Paleo diet, but you will need to follow some guidelines.

Beware of Hidden Fat and Sugar

Ready-to-eat Paleo products can be useful for those who choose to live gluten-free, but it is important to read food labels carefully to see exactly what you're eating. Gluten-free processed foods, such as cookies, crackers, breads, cereals and desserts, present some of the same problems that low-fat and nonfat products did when they became popular. Many people felt cheated or tricked when they found out that some of these products had more sugar and calories than the full-fat versions. Similarly, many gluten-free processed foods contain a great deal of both sugar and fat to enhance taste and improve texture.

Watch Out for Overeating

It's easy to unintentionally eat too much of foods that we perceive as being healthy. You may have run into this problem when "100-calorie" snack packets hit the shelves, or when you found out that healthy smoothies were packed with calories and needed to be eaten as a treat rather than a daily staple. Many of us believe more is better and eat more in general. Some studies have shown that overeating alone can account for the obesity epidemic in America.

Be Sure to Eat Frequently

Skipping meals lowers your blood sugar and raises your insulin levels. This creates cravings for quick-fix carbohydrates, which you're probably used to getting from things like cereal, bread, fruit and grain bars, cookies and other foods made from the easily absorbed carbohydrates contained in grains.

If you skip meals, you'll be setting yourself up for either eating something that will hurt you (if you have celiac disease or gluten sensitivity), or eating something that's just not good for you — and certainly not good for weight loss, like a soda or candy bar.

By eating at least every two hours or so, you can avoid many of these carbohydrate cravings and increase your chances of losing weight on a gluten-free diet.

Get Plenty of Fiber

If you've been getting most of your fiber from healthy, whole-grain cereals and breads, you're going to need to increase your plant fiber intake. Overall, plant fiber has been shown to be a healthier fiber choice than the fiber from grains.

Be sure to eat plenty of the most fibrous fruits and vegetables, including apples, mangoes, papaya, broccoli, Brussels sprouts and celery. Plant foods contain soluble (dissolves in water) and insoluble (doesn't dissolve in water) fiber, and both are real powerhouses. As long as you eat a wide variety of fresh fruits and vegetables daily, you'll keep your fiber intake at a healthy level. If you're one of those people who have trouble getting enough fruits and veggies, consider adding psyllium husk to smoothies, shakes, baked goods and even scrambled eggs.

Get Plenty of Protein

Breads, pasta and cereals make up a huge chunk of the daily calories most Americans eat. If you cut them from your diet and don't replace them with Paleo options, you're likely to cut your calories way down, too.

If you find yourself feeling hungry frequently, take a look at your calorie intake and make sure you're eating enough. Protein will help you feel satisfied. Make sure you eat plenty of healthy protein, such as lean meats, fish, shellfish, eggs and dairy (if you can have it). You'll increase calories in a healthy way and the protein will make you feel full longer than the empty calories of fats or carbohydrates.

Drink Plenty of Water

Dieters get tired of hearing about how they need to drink plenty of water, but water aids digestion, helps you feel full and even helps your body get rid of excess stored fat. Going Paleo means changes to your digestive system — changes that will be helped along by getting adequate water (64 ounces a day — more if you work out or spend much time outdoors).

Don't be discouraged or assume that your weight loss goals will have to be put on hold if you go on a Paleo diet. As long as you follow these guidelines, eat sensibly and get plenty of exercise, you can lose weight on a Paleo diet.

2. Paleo Diet Basics

Knowing What You Can Eat and What You Cannot

This is the most important part of going paleo. A gluten-free diet isn't as simple as going vegetarian or even going on a raw-food diet. Gluten is in so many products and comes in so many forms that reading labels is essential.

Knowing How to Replace the Foods You Cannot Have

It's easy and very common to get discouraged and upset when you think you can never again have chocolate cake, a blueberry muffin or a hearty sandwich. Fortunately, going Paleo in the real world means you can have your cake and eat it too.

Knowing How to Eat No Matter Where You Are

Most people don't have the option of going Paelo in a bubble — nor would we want to. We eat in restaurants, at the homes of friends and on food-centered holidays.

Have Plenty of Choices, No Matter How Busy You Are, How Little You Cook or How Tight Your Budget Is

Some of us love to cook and have plenty of time to spend doing it. Others are on very tight schedules or just don't enjoy spending much time in the kitchen.

Gluten-free packaged foods can be expensive, especially if you're also buying traditional versions for the rest of the family. If you're on a tight grocery budget, you can save a great deal of money by using the recipes here and many others to prepare your own gluten-free foods at home — at a fraction of the cost.

Going Paelo isn't necessarily simple, and it definitely

isn't without compromise. But going Paleo in the real world can be delicious, affordable and easier than you think.

Foods You Might Not Realize Have Gluten

As you'll see later in the Not Allowed Foods List, gluten is in a lot of food products that don't come to mind when you're thinking about wheat, barley, rye and their byproducts. For instance, many types of vinegar are made of malt, which is a barley product. Now you know to avoid malt vinegar, but many salad dressings, barbecue sauces and steak sauces will list vinegar on their ingredients list without telling you what kind of vinegar.

Many soy sauces contain gluten as well. Condiments are a tricky group overall. Many commercial mayonnaises use gluten as a binder and stabilizer. Some mustards contain gluten as well. Tomato sauces sometimes contain gluten, and tomato paste often does. These items can show up in commercial ketchups, spaghetti sauces and barbecue sauces. The problem is that only "tomato paste" is listed in the ingredients.

Part of the issue with hidden gluten is that it can be used in the packaging or processing of a product, too, without it actually being considered an ingredient. For instance, some gums are dusted with wheat and other flours to keep them from being sticky. Candy bars may be made without gluten, but the conveyor belts on which they are processed are often dusted with wheat flour.

Yeast may be either grown or dried on wheat. Wheat is sometimes added to ice cream to prevent the formation of ice crystals. There may be wheat flour in your spices, too, particularly spice blends like Cajun or Italian seasonings. Crispy rice cereals and many corn cereals often contain wheat, as can yogurt, lunch meat and even some packages of ground beef. Even your shortening may contain vitamin E that was extracted from wheat.

Your best defense is to keep your foods lists with you when you're ordering food online or buying groceries in the supermarket.

Gluten Is Present in Nonfood Items Too

If you're feeling overwhelmed by the vast number of food items that may contain gluten, you probably don't want to hear that it's present in a lot of inedible products too. Unfortunately, you need to be just as aware of these.

For those with celiac disease and gluten sensitivity, household items can present just as much danger as a slice of Wonder Bread. Those going gluten-free voluntarily don't need to worry about these products so much, but even very slight amounts of gluten are dangerous to people with celiac disease, gluten sensitivity or a wheat allergy.

One of the groups of household products that often contains gluten is glues and adhesives. Many brands and forms of glue and paste contain gluten, as can postage stamps, stickers and the adhesive on envelopes.

Art supplies such as paints, Play-Doh and clay often

contain flour. If your child has been diagnosed with celiac disease or gluten sensitivity, be sure to check their art supplies and notify their teacher as well. You also want to check the glue, paste and stickers you have in your home. Even if your child has no problem with gluten, if you or another adult does, you'll need to take precautions. It may be best to toss what you already have and start over with products you know are gluten-free.

Cleaning agents can also contain gluten, especially dish soap, dishwasher detergent and "soft" cleansers and bar soaps. Gloves may be the answer, but latex and household gloves are often dusted with flour to make them easier to put on and remove. You can order undusted gloves from a medical supply store or find them in many drugstores. They're very inexpensive and disposable, and come in boxes of fifty or one hundred. Even if you don't usually wear gloves to wash dishes or clean the house, they're good to have if your family is not gluten-free and you'll be handling foods with gluten.

Toiletries are also a concern, especially since you have a decent chance of ingesting them by getting them on your hands and then putting your fingers on or in your mouth. These include shampoos, conditioners, lotions, facial cleansers, sun protection products, lipsticks and lip balms, and even toothpaste and mouthwash.

Again, your best defense is to call or e-mail the major manufacturers or look for a contact number on the products you already have in your house. They can usually find out for you whether the product you're using is gluten-free.

About Substitutes

For people who can't have gluten, baked goods are often a source of disappointment instead of the enjoyable indulgence they are meant to be. The typical flours used for baking and cooking include rye, barley and wheat flours, all of which have at least a small amount of gluten. Fortunately, there are several good flour alternatives you can use to turn that cake, bread or pastry into a delicious, gluten-free dessert that even your family will enjoy. Before I get into substitutions, though, there are a couple of tips you need to know that will help your baked goods turn out better.

Guar Gum or Xanthan Gum Help With Rise and Texture

In addition to trapping air in baked goods and making them rise well, gluten acts as a binding and emulsifying agent. In other words, it helps hold together and even disperse all the ingredients in a batter or dough. Therefore, when you remove gluten, your end product may be crumbly or grainy. A good way to help with this problem is to add one teaspoon of guar gum or xanthan gum per cup of gluten-free flour. This helps with binding and will produce a smoother texture. Measure carefully though, because if you use too much, the end product may turn out heavy or gummy.

Now let's look at some good gluten-free substitutes for your favorite flours.

Good Flours for Baking

Because different flours interact differently with the other ingredients in a recipe, some gluten-free flours are more suited to baking than others.

It's best if you experiment and find your own preferred blends, but when you substitute flours in your favorite traditional recipes, use the following measurements per cup of wheat flour.

Tapioca flour: Substitute tapioca cup for cup with wheat flour. Use 1 cup tapioca for every 1 ¼ cups barley flour or 1 ⅓ cups rye flour.

Sorghum flour: Perhaps the best-tasting flour, this should be used in equal amounts when substituting for wheat, rye or barley flours.

Good Substitutes for Batter

If you want to batter fish, meats or vegetables to fry or bake them, some good substitutions include corn flour or rice flour mixed with ¼ teaspoon baking powder. Don't use guar gum or xanthan gum for batters; it's not necessary.

Good Gluten-Free Substitutions for Pancakes

Just about everybody loves pancakes, crepes and waffles for breakfast (or even for supper, for those of you who are a bit more unconventional), but people who need to go gluten-free usually have to skip them. Well, now you don't have to do that! Just substitute rice, sorghum or buckwheat flour in your pancake, crepe and waffle recipes.

Buckwheat flour is naturally gluten-free, but remember that it has a very distinctive flavor and texture. Also, make sure that when you buy it, it actually says "gluten-free," because buckwheat flour is frequently processed with the same machinery that processes wheat flour and may become contaminated. If you're making pancakes, crepes or waffles, you want them to rise, so remember to use guar gum or xanthan gum in your pancake batter, regardless of which gluten-free flour you're using.

Choosing the Best Flour for the Job

Here are a couple basic rules to use when trying to decide which flour to use.

Medium gluten-free flours, such as sorghum flour, are similar to using white, all-purpose flour.

Heavier gluten-free grain flours are similar to baking with whole-grain flours such as barley and rye.

When it comes right down to it, your choice of gluten-free flour substitutions is all about what tastes good to you. Experiment, try mixing the different flours and figure out what works best for your particular tastes. The fact that you can't have gluten doesn't mean you have to go without dessert or batter-fried foods. Also, several of the top prepackaged cake and dessert manufacturers now offer gluten-free options that taste great and are just as convenient to make as their gluten-containing cousins. Whatever you do though, don't think your cake and cookie days are over just because you can't have gluten.

3. The Paleo Lifestlye

Living with a food restriction is never easy, but when you're trying to coordinate a tasty meal that everybody in the house can eat, it gets even tougher. Because so many things contain gluten, you need to be extremely careful about the ingredients you use. Fortunately, there are many options available to you that are both gluten-free and delicious. Soon you'll be making every meal a delight for the entire family without sacrificing taste or leaving anybody out.

Plan Your Meals Ahead

This is probably the easiest thing you can do to make meal preparation easier. If you typically make spaghetti for the family on Tuesday, make gluten-free noodles to top with gluten-free spaghetti sauce instead. If your clan has requested your special fried chicken over the weekend, you can make sure you have enough roast chicken for yourself and eat the same non-gluten side dishes as the rest of the family.

When you plan ahead it's easier to avoid cooking two whole separate meals.

Keep Gluten-Free Goodies at Home

There's no reason everyone has to go without goodies just because one person has a gluten restriction. It's okay to keep cookies, cakes and breads in the house, but try to have substitutes for the person who is going gluten-free. There are many good prepackaged desserts, cookies and snacks that are both gluten-free and delicious, so keep some of these on hand so that nobody feels left out at snack time. Remember to mark all gluten-free foods with a big "GF" or other recognizable mark so that it's obvious the food is okay to eat.

Take a Course on Gluten-Free Cooking

Expanding your repertoire of gluten-free recipes will make it easier for you to prepare gluten-free meals the whole family will love. This will save you the time and trouble of making something different for yourself.

It's also a great way to get out and meet other people and exchange ideas with those who share your challenges. By taking a course at a community college or culinary school, you'll not only learn some new techniques, but will also be able to network with other people and learn even more ways to make your life easier. Check with your local community college, because often, if there isn't an adult education course available on a given subject, they may be willing to create one if there's enough interest.

Teach Other Family Members About the Diet

It's important that everybody in the family understands the ins and outs of a Paleo diet. They should also know why it's so important that mom, dad, brother or sister not eat gluten, so that they will take the situation as seriously as they should. Also, be positive about it. If your child is the one with the gluten issue, they'll be learning how to deal with this restriction from you. Be sure you approach this as just another part of daily life — important, yes, but not something that should make them feel ostracized or different.

Be Willing to Experiment

There are many tasty options out there for baking and cooking that are gluten-free. Quinoa, buckwheat flour and corn flour are all delicious as well as healthy. By experimenting with different flavors, you'll find out what works and what doesn't. As you find good recipes, be sure to save them so you can make them again. This will also make it easier for someone else to cook gluten-free for you!

Double or Triple Up When You Cook

The hardest, most time-consuming part of cooking anything, whether it's gluten-free or not, is the preparation. If you're taking the time to cook on the weekends or on your nights off, just double up the recipes. Then all you have to do is pop the leftovers in the oven or microwave and you have an awesome, homemade meal in just a few minutes.

Gluten-free pancakes or waffles can also be made ahead of time. These are both great bread substitutes when making a sandwich and are easy for a younger child to prepare on their own. A few moments in the microwave or toaster and they have either an instant meal or a base for their sandwich.

Strategies for Eating at Restaurants, at Parties and on Holidays

The hardest time to follow any diet may be during special occasions. By planning ahead and using these tips, you'll be able to make it through the pitfalls of a gluten-riddled environment safely, happily and with a full belly.

Educate Yourself

As with any diet, you need to know what you can have and what you can't. Because gluten is used so widely in everything from breads to gravies and sauces, it's important that you know what foods it may be in. By educating yourself in advance, you can easily pick out menu items that are likely to be safe and then ask the server about them before you order.

Ask for the Gluten-Free Menu

Because of the prevalence of people who can't have gluten, many restaurants now offer a gluten-free menu — so ask for it. Check out the restaurant on the Internet beforehand to see if it mentions gluten-free options. At the very least, many restaurants have their menus posted online so that you can figure out in advance what you want to order.

If all else fails, let the server know that you have can't have gluten and choose a couple of menu items for them to ask the chef about. Restaurants are generally willing to accommodate special dietary needs, so if there's a particular item that you really want, the chef may very well make you a version of it that's gluten-free. Just be sure the kitchen knows how to safely prepare gluten-free dishes without danger of cross-contamination. For instance, that means no wiping down plates with towels that have touched sauces or gravies with gluten.

Alert Your Hosts in Advance

If your host knows in advance that you or a member of your party can't have gluten, they can make sure to include a few gluten-free foods. If you're not comfortable letting them know, make sure that you either eat before you go or take something appropriate with you.

If it's a catered party or function, you have options there, too. Many caterers specifically ask the host if there are any special dietary needs when they are discussing and planning meals. They will gladly prepare something you can have, so that you may enjoy eating with everybody else without worry. Remember, a good host wants to meet the needs of their guests and may feel bad if you don't let them know in advance so that they can be prepared.

Teach Your Child About Eating Gluten-Free

When it comes right down to it, it's your responsibility to make sure your child knows what foods are safe to eat. Until they can learn what is and is not okay, you'll need to teach them not to eat anything without asking you first. A good alternative is to teach them what foods are acceptable to eat anytime you're out, such as vegetables and fruits, and which foods they need to either skip or ask you about. If there are snacks or appetizers placed on a buffet, take your child to the table and explain what they can have.

Take Safe Foods With You

If you don't feel comfortable telling the host about your needs, or if you're not sure there are going to be foods available for you or your child, take something with you. This way, you know for a fact that the food is safe. This is a good idea, especially if you're going on a picnic or to an outing that's just going to have snacks.

If you're the one with the gluten allergy, you can just eat before you go, but if it's your child with the restriction, make sure you take something so that they aren't left out in case there's nothing gluten-free available. One nice thing about taking a gluten-free dish along: Other guests may be coming who also have gluten issues. Your dish might save the occasion for them, too.

Plan Ahead

If you're throwing a party or cooking the holiday meal, plan your menu in advance, down to the last ingredient. There's nothing worse than being ready to mash the potatoes and realizing that you didn't get any gluten-free broth with which to make the gravy. A little bit of planning will make your life much easier, so take the extra time to do it right.

Living a Paleo lifestyle isn't always easy when you're trying to do it on the go. On top of the regular stress created by just attending a party or getting the kids ready to go out, you also have to worry about whether or not there are going to be safe foods available for you or your family member. By educating yourself and planning ahead, you can take much of the stress out of the ordeal and turn it instead into the happy event that it should be.

Foods You Can and Cannot Eat

I've provided lists of Allowed and Not Allowed Foods and ingredients in the next section. The lists may be cumbersome, but they'll help you to check ingredient labels as you do your shopping.

Allowed Foods List

Acacia gum

Acesulfame potassium (aka Acesulfame K)

Acetanisole

Acetophenone

Acorn quercus

Adipic acid

Adzuki bean

Agar

Agave

Albumen

Alcohol (distilled spirits, including bourbon, gin, rum, Scotch whiskey, tequila, vodka)

Alfalfa

Algae

Algin

Alginate

Alginic acid

Alkalized cocoa

Allicin

Almond nut

Alpha-amylase

Alpha-lactalbumin

Aluminum

Amaranth

Ambergris

Ammonium hydroxide

Ammonium phosphate

Ammonium sulphate

Amylopectin

Amylose

Annatto

Annatto color

Apple cider vinegar

Arabic gum

Arrowroot

Artichokes

Artificial butter flavor

Artificial flavoring

Ascorbic acid

Aspartame (may cause irritable bowel syndrome symptoms)

Aspartic acid

Aspic

Astragalus gummifer

Autolyzed yeast extract

Avena sativia (if allowed oats)

Avena sativia extract (if allowed oats)

Avidin

Azodicarbonamide

Baking soda

Balsamic vinegar

Bean, adzuki

Bean, hyacinth

Bean, lentil

Bean, mung

Bean, romano (borlotti)

Bean, tepary

Beans

Beeswax

Benzoic acid

Besan (chickpea flour)

Beta carotene

Beta glucan (if allowed oats)

Betaine

BHA

BHT

Bicarbonate of soda

Biotin

Blue cheese

Brown sugar

Buckwheat

Butter (check additives)

Butyl compounds

Butylated hydroxyanisole

Calcium acetate

Calcium carbonate

Calcium caseinate

Calcium chloride

Calcium disodium

Calcium hydroxide

Calcium lactate

Calcium pantothenate

Calcium phosphate

Calcium propionate

Calcium silicate

Calcium sorbate

Calcium stearate

Calcium stearoyl lactylate

Calcium sulfate

Calrose

Camphor

Cane sugar

Cane vinegar

Canola (rapeseed)

Canola oil (rapeseed oil)

Caprylic acid

Carageenan chondrus crispus

Carbonated water

Carboxymethyl cellulose

Carmine

Carnauba wax

Carob bean

Carob bean gum

Carob flour

Carrageenan

Casein

Cassava manihot esculenta

Castor oil

Catalase

Cellulose[1]

Cellulose ether

Cellulose gum

Cetyl alcohol

Cetyl stearyl alcohol

Champagne vinegar

Chana (chickpea)

Chana flour (chickpea flour)

Cheeses (most, but check ingredients)

Chestnuts

Chickpea (garbanzo beans)

Chlorella

Chocolate

Chocolate liquor

Choline chloride

Chromium citrate

Chymosin

Cider

Citric acid

Citrus red No. 2

Cochineal

Cocoa

Cocoa butter

Coconut

Coconut vinegar

Collagen

Colloidal silicon dioxide

Confectioners' glaze

Copernicia cerifera

Copper sulphate

Corn

Corn flour

Corn gluten

Corn masa flour

Corn meal

Corn starch

Corn sugar

Corn sugar vinegar

Corn sweetener

Corn syrup

Corn syrup solids

Corn vinegar

Cortisone

Cotton seed

Cotton seed oil

Cowitch

Cowpea

Cream of tartar

Crospovidone

Curds

Cyanocobalamin

Cysteine

Dal (lentils)

D-alpha-tocopherol

Dasheen flour (taro)

Dates

D-calcium pantothenate

Delactosed whey

Demineralized whey

Desamidocollagen

Dextran

Dextrose

Diglycerides

Dioctyl sodium

Dioctyl sodium solfosuccinate

Dipotassium phosphate

Disodium guanylate

Disodium inosinate

Disodium phosphate

Distilled alcohols

Distilled vinegar

Distilled white vinegar

Dutch processed cocoa

EDTA (ethylenediaminetetraacetic acid)

Egg

Egg yolk

Elastin

Ester gum

Ethyl alcohol

Ethyl maltol

Ethyl vanillin

Ethylenediaminetetraacetic acid

Expeller pressed canola oil

FD&C blue No. 1 dye

FD&C blue No. 1 lake

FD&C blue No. 2 dye

FD&C blue No. 2 lake

FD&C green No. 3 dye

FD&C green No. 3 lake

FD&C red No. 3 dye

FD&C red No. 40 dye

FD&C red No. 40 lake

FD&C yellow No. 5 dye

FD&C yellow No. 6 dye

FD&C yellow No. 6 lake

Ferric orthophosphate

Ferrous fumerate

Ferrous gluconate

Ferrous lactate

Ferrous sulfate

Fish (fresh)

Flax

Folacin

Folate

Folic acid–folacin

Formaldehyde

Fructose

Fruit (including dried)

Fruit vinegar

Fumaric acid

Galactose

Garbanzo beans

Gelatin

Glucoamylase

Gluconolactone

Glucose

Glucose syrup

Glutamate (free)

Glutamic acid

Glutamine (amino acid)

Glycerides

Glycerin

Glycerol monooleate

Glycol

Glycol monosterate

Glycolic acid

Gram flour (chickpea)

Grape skin extract

Grits, corn

Guar gum

Gum arabic

Gum base

Gum tragacanth

Gum, acacia

Hemp

Hemp seeds

Herb vinegar

Herbs

Hexanedioic acid

High fructose corn syrup

Hominy

Honey

Hops

Horseradish (pure)

Hyacinth bean

Hydrogen peroxide

Hydrolyzed caseinate

Hydrolyzed meat protein

Hydrolyzed soy protein

Hydroxypropyl cellulose

Hydroxypropyl methylcellulose

Hypromellose

Illepe

Inulin

Invert sugar

Iodine

Iron ammonium citrate

Isinglass

Isolated soy protein

Isomalt

Job's tears

Jowar (sorghum)

Karaya gum

Kasha (roasted buckwheat)

K-carmine color

Keratin

K-gelatin

Kudzu

Kudzu root starch

Lactalbumin phosphate

Lactase

Lactic acid

Lactitol

Lactose

Lactulose

Lanolin

Lard

L-cysteine

Lecithin

Lemon grass

Lentils

Licorice

Licorice extract

Lipase

L-leucine

L-lysine

L-methionine

Locust bean gum

L-tryptophan

Magnesium carbonate

Magnesium hydroxide

Magnesium oxide

Maize

Maize, waxy

Malic acid

Malt dextrin

Maltol

Manganese sulfate

Manioc

Masa

Masa farina

Masa flour

Meat (fresh)

Medium chain triglycerides

Menhaden oil

Methyl cellulose[2]

Microcrystalline cellulose

Micro-particulated egg white protein

Milk

Milk protein isolate

Millet

Milo (sorghum)

Mineral oil

Mineral salts

Molybdenum amino acid chelate

Mono and diglycerides

Monocalcium phosphate

Monoglycerides

Monopotassium phosphate

Monosaccharides

Monosodium glutamate (MSG)

Monosterate

MSG

Mung bean

Musk

Mustard flour

Myristic acid

Natural smoke flavor

Neotame

Niacin

Niacin–niacin amide

Nitrates

Nitrous oxide

Nonfat milk

Nut, acorn

Nut, almond

Nuts (except wheat, rye and barley)

Oats (only if allowed)

Oils and fats

Oleic acid

Oleoresin

Olestra

Oleyl alcohol

Oleyl oil

Orange B

Oryzanol

Palmitic acid

Pantothenic acid

Papain

Paprika

Paraffin

Partially hydrogenated cottonseed oil

Partially hydrogenated soybean oil

Pea flour

Pea starch

Pea, cow

Peanut flour

Peanuts

Peas

Pectin

Pectinase

Peppermint oil

Peppers

Pepsin

Peru balsam

Petrolatum

PGPR (polyglycerol polyricinoleate)

Phenylalanine

Phosphoric acid

Phosphoric glycol

Pigeon peas

Polenta

Polydextrose

Polyethylene glycol

Polyglycerol

Polyglycerol polyricinoleate (PGPR)

Polysorbate 60

Polysorbate 80

Polysorbates

Potassium benzoate

Potassium caseinate

Potassium citrate

Potassium iodide

Potassium lactate

Potassium matabisulphite

Potassium sorbate

Potato flour

Potato starch

Potatoes

Povidone

Prinus

Pristane

Propolis

Propyl gallate

Propylene glycol

Propylene glycol monosterate

Protease

Psyllium

Pyridoxine hydrochloride

Quinoa

Ragi

Raisin vinegar

Rape

Recaldent

Reduced iron

Rennet

Rennet casein

Resinous glaze

Reticulin

Riboflavin

Rosin

Royal jelly

Saccharin

Saffron

Sago

Sago flour

Sago palm

Sago starch

Saifun (bean threads)

Salt

Seaweed

Seed, sesame

Seed, sunflower

Seeds (except wheat, rye and barley)

Shea

Sherry vinegar

Silicon dioxide

Soba (be sure it's 100 percent buckwheat)

Sodium acetate

Sodium acid pyrophosphate

Sodium alginate

Sodium ascorbate

Sodium benzoate

Sodium caseinate

Sodium citrate

Sodium erythrobate

Sodium hexametaphosphate

Sodium lactate

Sodium lauryl sulfate

Sodium meta-bisulphite

Sodium nitrate

Sodium phosphate

Sodium polyphosphate

Sodium silaco aluminate

Sodium stannate

Sodium stearoyl lactylate

Sodium sulphite

Sodium tripolyphosphate

Solfosuccinate

Sorbic acid

Sorbitan monosterate

Sorbitol, mannitol (may cause irritable bowl syndrome symptoms)

Sorghum

Sorghum flour

Soy

Soy lecithin

Soy protein

Soy protein isolate

Soybean

Spices (pure)

Spirits (distilled, without malt or barley)

Spirit vinegar

Stearamide

Stearamine

Stearates

Stearic acid

Stearyl lactate

Stevia

Succotash (corn and beans)

Sucralose

Sucrose

Sulfites

Sulfur dioxide

Sunflower seed

Sweet chestnut flour

Tagatose

Tallow

Tapioca

Tapioca flour

Tapioca starch

Tara gum

Taro

Taro gum

Taro root

Tartaric acid

Tartrazine

TBHQ (tetra or tributylhydroquinone)

Tea

Tea-tree oil

Teff

Teff flour

Tepary bean

Textured vegetable protein

Thiamine hydrochloride

Thiamine mononitrate

Thiamin hydrochloride

Titanium dioxide

Tofu (soybean curd)

Torula yeast

Tragacanth

Tragacanth gum

Triacetin

Tri-calcium phosphate

Trypsin

Turmeric (kurkuma)

TVP

Tyrosine

Urad/urid beans

Urad/urid dal (peas)

Urad/urid flour

Vanilla extract

Vanilla flavoring

Vanillin

Vinegar (all except malt)

Vinegars (distilled)

Vitamin A (retinol)

Vitamin A palmitate

Vitamin B1

Vitamin B-12

Vitamin B2

Vitamin B6

Vitamin D

Vitamin E acetate

Waxy maize

Whey

Whey protein concentrate

Whey protein isolate

White vinegar

Wild rice

Wine (and grape-based fermented beverages, such as champagne)

Wine vinegars (distilled)

Xanthan gum

Xylitol

Yam flour

Yeast

Yogurt (plain, unflavored)

Zinc oxide

Zinc sulfate

[1] The problem with caramel color is it may or may not contain gluten, depending on how it is manufactured.

[2] If this ingredient is made in North America, it is likely to be gluten-free.

Not Allowed Foods

Abyssinian hard wheat (Triticum durum)

Alcohol (non-distilled, malt beverages, rye whiskey)

Amp-isostearoyl hydrolyzed wheat protein

Atta flour

Barley grass (may contain seeds)

Barley hordeum vulgare

Barley malt

Beer (most contain barley or wheat)

Bleached flour

Bran

Bread flour

Brewer's yeast

Brown flour

Bulgur (bulgur wheat, nuts)

Bulgur wheat

Cereal binding

Chilton

Club wheat (Triticum aestivum subspecies compactum)

Common wheat (Triticum aestivum)

Cookie crumbs

Cookie dough

Cookie dough pieces

Couscous

Crisped rice

Dinkle (spelt)

Disodium oleamido peg-2 solfosuccinate

Durum wheat (Triticum durum)

Edible coatings

Edible films

Edible starch

Einkorn (Triticum monococcum)

Emmer (Triticum dicoccon)

Enriched bleached flour

Enriched bleached wheat flour

Enriched flour

Farina

Farina graham

Faro

Filler

Flour (normally this is wheat)

Fu (dried wheat gluten)

Germ

Graham flour

Granary flour

Groats (barley, wheat)

Hard wheat

Heeng

Hing

Hordeum vulgare extract

Hydrolyzed wheat gluten

Hydrolyzed wheat protein

Hydrolyzed wheat starch

Hydroxypropyltrimonium hydrolyzed wheat protein

Kamet (wheat pasta)

Kecap manis (soy sauce)

Ketjap manis (soy sauce)

Kluski pasta

Macha wheat (Triticum aestivum)

Maida (Indian wheat flour)

Malt

Malt extract

Malt flavoring

Malt syrup

Malt vinegar

Malted barley flour

Malted milk

Matza, matzah, matzo

Matzo meal

Matzo semolina

Meringue

Meripro 711

Mir

Nishasta

Oriental wheat (Triticum turanicum)

Orzo pasta

Pasta (made with not allowed flours)

Pearl barley

Persian wheat (Triticum carthlicum)

Perungayam

Polish wheat (Triticum polonicum)

Poulard wheat (Triticum turgidum)

Rice malt (if barley or koji are used)

Roux

Rusk

Rye

Seitan

Semolina

Semolina triticum

Shot wheat (Triticum aestivum)

Small spelt

Spelt (Triticum spelta)

Spirits (non-distilled)

Sprouted wheat or barley

Stearyldimonium hydroxypropyl hydrolyzed wheat protein

Strong flour

Suet in packets

Tabbouleh

Tabouli

Teriyaki sauce

Timopheevii wheat (Triticum timopheevii)

Triticale x triticosecale

Triticum vulgare (wheat) flour lipids

Triticum vulgare (wheat) germ extract

Triticum vulgare (wheat) germ oil

Udon (wheat noodles)

Unbleached flour

Vavilovi wheat (Triticum aestivum)

Vital wheat gluten

Wheat (Triticum vulgare) bran extract

Wheat amino acids

Wheat bran extract

Wheat germ extract

Wheat germ glycerides

Wheat germ oil

Wheat germ, amidopropyldimonium hydroxypropyl hydrolyzed wheat protein

Wheat grass (may contain seeds)

Wheat nuts

Wheat protein

Wheat, Abyssinian hard (Triticum durum)

Wheat, bulgur

Wheat (Durum triticum)

Wheat (Triticum aestivum)

Wheat (Triticum monococcum)

Whole-meal flour

Wild einkorn (Triticum boeotictim)

Wild emmer (Triticum dicoccoides)

Foods That Require Caution

The following items may or may not contain gluten, depending on where and how they are made. It is sometimes necessary to check with the manufacturer to find out.

Artificial color[3]
Baking powder[3]
Caramel color[1,2]
Caramel flavoring[1,2]
Clarifying agents[3]
Coloring[3]
Dextrimaltose[1,6]
Dextrins[1,6]
Dry-roasted nuts[3]
Emulsifiers[3]
Enzymes[3]
Fat replacer[3]
Flavoring[5]

Food starch modified[1,3]

Food starch[1,3]

Glucose syrup[3]

Gravy cubes[3]

Ground spices[3]

HPP[4]

HVP[4]

Hydrogenated starch hydrolysate[3]

Hydrolyzed plant protein[3]

Hydrolyzed protein[3]

Hydrolyzed vegetable protein[3]

Hydroxy-propylated starch[3]

Maltose[3]

Miso[3]

Mixed tocopherols[3]

Modified food starch[1,3]

Modified starch[1,3]

Natural flavoring[5]

Natural flavors[5]

Natural juices[3]

Non-dairy creamer[3]

Pre-gelatinized starch[3]

Protein hydrolysates[3]

Seafood analogs[3]

Seasonings[3]

Sirimi[3]

Smoke flavoring[3]

Soba noodles[3]

Soy sauce solids[3]

Soy sauce[3]

Sphingolipids[3]

Stabilizers[3]

Starch[1,3]

Stock cubes[3]

Suet[4]

Tocopherols[3]

Vegetable broth[3]

Vegetable gum[3]

Vegetable protein[3]

Vegetable starch[3]

Vitamins[3]

Wheat starch[4]

[1] If this ingredient is made in North America, it is likely to be gluten-free.

[2] The problem with caramel color is it may or may not contain gluten, depending on how it is manufactured.

[3] May use a grain or byproduct containing gluten in the

manufacturing process, or as an ingredient.

[4] Most celiac disease support organizations in the United States and Canada do not believe that wheat starch is safe for people with celiac disease. In Europe, however, most doctors and celiac disease support organizations consider Codex Alimentarius Quality wheat starch acceptable in the celiac diet. This is a higher quality of wheat starch than is generally available in the United States or Canada.

[5] According to 21 CFR, Section 101.22: "The term natural flavor or natural flavoring means the essential oil, oleoresin, essence or extractive, protein hydrolysate, distillate, or any product of roasting, heating or enzymolysis, which contains the flavoring constituents derived from a spice, fruit or fruit juice, vegetable or vegetable juice, edible yeast, herb, bark, bud, root, leaf or similar plant material, meat, seafood, poultry, eggs, dairy products, or fermentation products thereof, whose significant function in food is flavoring rather than nutritional."

[6] Dextrin is an incompletely hydrolyzed starch. It is prepared by dry-heating corn, waxy maize, waxy milo, potato, arrowroot, wheat, rice, tapioca, or sago

starches, or by dry-heating the starches after treatment with safe and suitable alkalis, acids, or pH control agents, and drying the acid- or alkali-treated starch. Therefore, unless you know the source, you must avoid dextrin.

4. Shopping Tips

Grocery shopping can be a real chore when you're on a Paleo diet, especially when you're first starting out. There can be a lot of new things to learn and to buy. Be prepared to take more time shopping, and also try to remember that in a short time you will learn which brands and products are safe to buy and be able to shop almost as quickly, if not just as quickly, as you did before.

Follow these guidelines and hints to help you cover your bases and streamline your grocery shopping. Doing so will help make the process less stressful.

Make a Shopping Notebook

This is one of the very best steps you can take, and your notebook will become an invaluable tool. A notebook that has some pockets is best. An old agenda or Day Runner–type book is great, and one that fits in your handbag will be most convenient.

Decide Where You're Going to Do Your Shopping

Most supermarkets have a Paleo section in addition to the gluten-free products spread throughout the store. Some grocery stores, particularly health food stores, tend to have a wider selection. If running to more than one store is a hassle, consider ordering your gluten-free products from one of the online retailers in the resource guide and going to the supermarket only for fresh foods or foods that don't normally contain gluten anyway.

Check your supermarket's website to see if they have a list of Paleo products they stock. Many stores offer these lists online as a service to their customers. If they don't have one on their website, ask the manager next time you shop. If your store has a list of gluten-free products, keep it in your notebook.

Make a Menu for the Week

Try to make a menu consisting mostly of recipes that use whole, fresh foods like meats, fresh seafood and fresh produce. This will allow for more flexibility in your menu planning. You'll also save money by not having to purchase a long list of gluten-free specialty products.

Make a Grocery List

Use the weekly menu as your guide. See what ingredients you need to purchase to make those meals and add them to your list.

Now, organize your shopping list. Some people like alphabetical lists, while others prefer to sort their lists by category and still others arrange their lists by grocery store aisle. Do what works for you, but definitely take the time to make a list. You can even create a master list and print several copies to save rewriting everything each week.

Keep your grocery list in your notebook. Having the list on hand will save you time and aggravation.

Keep It Fresh to Keep It Fast

Fresh meats, seafood and produce should be your staples. They don't require reading the labels (except possibly for ground beef) and they're better for you. The more you buy of these ingredients, the less time and money you'll have to spend in the packaged food sections.

Beat the Crowds

Try to pick a day and time to go shopping that is not as crowded. This will help balance out the extra time you'll spend reading labels. And if you have a question about gluten-free options, you may be more likely to find someone in the store who can help.

Make It Easy for Yourself

Shopping every one or two weeks is usually more economical and convenient, but is only possible if you plan ahead. If you are not the type to plan ahead, you may have to shop more frequently.

5. Paleo Meal Plans

The best meal plan for you will depend on several things, such as the time you have to spend cooking and whether you need to lose weight while on the Paleo diet.

I've provided different meal plans to use as a starting point to create your own menus and divided them into:

A meal plan for the Paleo cook

A meal plan for people with busy schedules

A meal plan for losing weight on a Paleo diet

A Meal Plan for the Paleo Cook

Breakfast

1 Morning Burrito

1 sliced mango

Coffee or tea

Morning Snack

1 stick mozzarella string cheese

1 fresh orange

Lunch

Tuna Stuffed Avocado

Tea or juice

Afternoon Snack

1 fresh apple

Dinner

Meat Loaf

Roasted asparagus with lemon pepper

Dessert

1 Brownie

A Meal Plan for People With Busy Schedules

Breakfast

½ cup gluten-free oats with blueberries and almond milk

Coffee or tea

1 banana

Morning Snack

1 fresh apple

1 stick mozzarella string cheese

Lunch

Turkey, tomato, spinach and gluten-free mayonnaise in a lettuce wrap

1 fresh orange

Juice or water

Afternoon Snack

6 gluten-free crackers

3 slices cheddar cheese

Dinner

Quick Fish Florentine

1 cup roasted carrots

Spinach salad with vinaigrette

1 gluten-free dinner roll

Juice or tea

Dessert

2 Chocolate Chip Cookies

A Meal Plan for Losing Weight on a Paleo Diet

Breakfast

½ cup gluten-free oats with almond milk

½ cup sliced fresh strawberries

1 hardboiled egg

Coffee or tea

Morning Snack

1 slice turkey breast rolled in 1 slice mozzarella

1 fresh peach

Lunch

Grilled chicken salad, made with 1 cup diced chicken breast, 1 cup fresh spinach, sliced tomato, sliced mushrooms

2 tablespoons light vinaigrette dressing

Water or tea

Afternoon Snack

1 sliced apple

1 tablespoon almond butter for dipping

Dinner

1 cup Lentil Garden Soup

Salad made with romaine lettuce, sliced red onion, diced red pepper

2 tablespoons light vinaigrette

Dessert

½ cup gluten-free sorbet or sherbet

6. Paleo Recipes

Breakfast

Melon, Mint and Cilantro Salad

2 tablespoons of chopped cilantro leaves
4 cups honeydew in 1-inch pieces
1 tablespoon of fresh lime juice
¼ cup of chopped fresh mint leaves
Honey to taste

In a large bowl, mix all ingredients. Toss to combine well. Refrigerate before serving, if desired.

Serves 2

Minty Apple & Grapefruit

1 teaspoon of finely chopped fresh mint

1 lime

2 pink grapefruits

2 sweet and firm apples

Honey to taste

Peel, core and slice apples and grapefruits. Add the slices in a bowl and gently stir. Squeeze lime. Add honey. Pour juice over fruit. Add fresh mint. Chill before serving.

Serves 2

Mushrooms and Pine Nuts Scrambled Eggs

2 eggs

2 tablespoons of finely chopped chives

½ cup of sliced mushrooms

1 tablespoon of Olive oil

1 tablespoon of pine nuts

Sea salt and pepper

Heat up oil in a frying pan with medium heat. Fry the mushrooms and chives for 3 to 4 minutes. Remove mixture from the pan.

Whisk eggs and add in the frying pan. Cook while stirring constantly. When eggs are almost cooked, add mushrooms and chives. Cook one minute longer. Add salt and pepper.

Serves 1

Nutty Peaches and Apples

2 apples, cored and chopped

2 peaches, chopped

½ cup of orange juice

1 cup of pecan halves

1 cup of walnuts

1 teaspoon of ground cinnamon

Add peaches and apples into an 8-inch square baking dish. Drizzle with orange juice and toss till fruit is well coated. In a food processor combine the walnuts, pecans and cinnamon, pulse till well combined. Spread mixture over the fruit to serve.

Serves 2

Omelet Blueberry Muffins

6 Eggs

30 blueberries

Sea salt and pepper

2 tablespoons of water

Olive oil for greasing

Prepare oven and heat it at 350 degrees

Fahrenheit. Grease a 6 cup muffin tray using olive oil.
Beat eggs in a large bowl. Add salt, pepper, water and
blueberry. Mix well. Add mixture into the muffin try.
Bake 20 minutes till a fork comes out clean.
Transfer muffins onto a plate. Serve with salsa if you
like.

Serves 6 muffins

Lunch

Baked Buffalo Wings

2 pounds of chicken wings

Salt and pepper

Sauce

3 tablespoons of coconut oil

3 tablespoons of white vinegar

½ teaspoon of cayenne pepper (optional)

½ teaspoon of hot (optional) paprika

1 teaspoon of garlic powder

1 teaspoon of onion powder

1 lemon or lime, juiced

1 teaspoon of sea salt

Preheat oven to 400 degrees Fahrenheit. Season wings with salt and pepper. Arrange wings as a single layer on a baking sheet and bake for 40-45 minutes. Melt coconut oil over medium heat in a medium sized saucepan, add garlic powder, onion powder, cayenne, paprika and salt and stir until evenly combined.

Add the juice from the lemon or lime and the vinegar. Turn off the heat and stir to mix well

Once the wings are done, heat up the sauce again and add wings to coat for a couple of minutes, or you can also pour the warm sauce into a large bowl add the wings and toss to coat.

Serve 2 pounds of wings

Baked Turkey & Mushrooms

4 ounces of sliced mushrooms

1 small boneless turkey breast, halved

1 tablespoon of olive oil

2 tablespoons of dried parsley flakes

½ teaspoon of dried tarragon

½ teaspoon of sea salt

A dash of pepper

¼ cup of white wine

2 tablespoons of coconut flour

¼ cup of cold water

Preheat oven at 400 degrees Fahrenheit

Place turkey breast halves into a baking dish with the skin side up. Brush them using olive oil and sprinkle with salt, pepper, parsley and tarragon. Add mushrooms on top and pour some wine.

Place the baking tray into the oven and bake for 30 minutes.

Remove turkey while keeping it warm.

Combine water and coconut flour in a saucepan till mixture gets smooth. Add cooking juices (from the baking dish) gradually and bring it to boil. Cook for 2 minutes while stirring constantly, till the sauce is thickened.

Serve turkey and mushrooms with sauce poured on top.

Serves 2

Basil Garlic &Tomato Salad

1 tomato

2 tablespoons of fresh basil

½ tablespoon of minced garlic

Sea salt and pepper

Half of a lettuce

Slice tomatoes into thin rounds. Mix basil, salt,

pepper, and garlic and spread mixture over the tomato slices. Set aside at room temperature for about 15 minutes so the flavors will be infused and serve on top of the lettuce leaves.

Serves 2

Carrot & Blueberries Salad

1 cup of blueberries

1 pound of carrots, peeled and shredded

1 cup of drained pineapple chunks

1 cup of 100% olive oil mayonnaise

2 tablespoons of honey

Combine all the ingredients in a bowl. Mix thoroughly and let them chill.

Serves 2

Carrot & Cilantro Soup

1 tablespoon of olive oil

1 small onion, chopped

½ teaspoon of crushed coriander seeds

½ pound of sliced carrots

2 cups of organic vegetable stock

½ cup of chopped fresh cilantro, and more for serving

Heat up olive oil in a large pan with medium heat. Add onion and coriander, cook for five minutes while stirring occasionally, till onions are softened but not browned. Add carrots. Cook covered for 15 to 20 minutes, while stirring from time to time.

Boil stock in a separate pot. Add carrot and onion mixture. Bring to boil again. Transfer mixture into a food processer. Blend till smooth. Use sea salt to season.

Return soup back to the pot. Add chopped cilantro and cook in low heat for about five minutes to allow the cilantro to infuse. Scoop the soup to warm bowls. Garnish with more cilantro.

Serves 2

Dinner

Apple Pork Chops

1 cup of fresh orange juice

Ground nutmeg

Ground cinnamon

2 pork chops with thick cut

1 teaspoon of olive oil

1 tablespoon of honey (optional)

Salt and pepper

1 tablespoon of almond butter

1 tart apple, peeled and sliced

2 tablespoons of chopped walnuts

Place a large skillet over medium-high heat. Brush the pork chops with olive oil. Place them in the hot skillet. Cover and let it cook for 5 to 6 minutes, while turning from time to time. Transfer chops to a plate.
Combine orange juice, nutmeg, cinnamon, salt, pepper and honey (if using) in a bowl. Add butter into the skillet. Stir in the mixture and apples. Cover and cook till apples are tender. Use a slotted spoon to transfer apples and arrange them on top of the pork chops.
Continue to cook the mixture uncovered, till the sauce is thickened. Add sauce over the chops and apples. Sprinkle with the chopped walnuts.

Serves 2

Baked Sea Bass

2 sea bass fillets

4 tablespoons of melted almond butter

1 tablespoon of lemon juice

½ cup of sliced mushroom

½ onion, finely chopped

Salt and pepper

Preheat oven to 350 degrees Fahrenheit.

In a bowl, combine lemon juice, melted butter, salt and pepper. Dip the fish fillet into the mixture and place fillets in a shallow baking pan. Top with mushrooms and onions. Spoon the remaining butter mixture over top.

Bake 15 minutes till the fish flakes.

Serves 2

Beef Brisket

1 pound of beef brisket

2 cups of boiling water

Dash of sea salt & pepper

Dash of garlic salt

1 tablespoon of vinegar

Dash of paprika

1 onion, sliced

Preheat oven at 350 degrees Fahrenheit. Place in oven and cook brisket uncovered in a pan for about 30 minutes. Add water, garlic salt, salt, vinegar, onion, pepper, paprika into the pan. Cover and roast in the oven for 30 more minutes till done. Remove the meat from the pan and cover with foil paper. Refrigerate overnight. Slice very thinly against the grain. Serve with juice.

Serves 2

Chicken & Avocado Soup

1 small chicken breast fillet

1 cube of chicken stock

2 cups of water

1 tablespoon of olive oil

1 small red onion, chopped nicely

1 teaspoon of ground cumin

½ teaspoon of chili powder

½ pound of diced tomatoes

1 large avocado, peeled, halved, and coarsely chopped

¼ cup of fresh coriander leaves, coarsely chopped

1 tablespoon of fresh lime juice

Place chicken and stock cube in a frying pan. Pour in the water and bring to simmer with low heat. Flip the chicken during the cooking. After cooked through, transfer chicken into a plate, while reserving the cooking liquid. Let chicken cool before you shred the meat.

Heat up oil in a saucepan with high heat. Add in onion to cook while stirring. Add chili and cumin and cook and stir for 30 seconds more. Add tomatoes and reserved liquid. Bring to boil. Add shredded chicken. Bring to boil. Reduce heat and simmer while stirring occasionally. Cook 10 minutes till the soup gets thickened. Season with salt and pepper

Combine avocado, lime juice and coriander. Ladle chicken soup into serving bowls and top with the avocado mixture. Serve.

Serves 2

Coconut Chicken Breast

1 tablespoon of olive oil

3 cloves of minced garlic

1 red onion, diced

4 small chicken breasts, boned, skinned, cut

into ½ inch pieces

> ½ cup of canned coconut milk
>
> 1 tablespoon of chopped fresh parsley

Sauce

1 garlic clove

¼ teaspoon of black pepper

¼ teaspoon of paprika

¼ cup of white vinegar

1 cup of water

1 small chicken bouillon cube

½ teaspoon of oregano

½ teaspoon of ground bay leaf

¼ cup of organic soy sauce or coconut aminos

1 tablespoon of honey

Sauté garlic and onion in a skillet. Add chicken breasts and brown lightly without burning the onions.
Combine sauce ingredients in a blender and blend, add into the skillet. Cover to simmer, while stirring occasionally, till the chicken is tender.
Pour coconut milk over the chicken, allowing it to simmer for 20 minutes more. Place on a serving dish. Ladle sauce over top. Use chopped parsley to

garnish.

Serves 2

Dessert

Apricot Brownie Cake

1 cup of almond butter

½ cup of honey

¼ cup of unsweetened cocoa powder

2 teaspoons of vanilla extract

¼ teaspoon of sea salt

½ teaspoon of baking soda

3 eggs

½ cup of fresh diced ripe apricots

Olive oil for greasing

Blend honey and almond butter till smooth. Add

the other ingredients and blend, with the exception of apricots. Add apricots to blended mix. Grease an 8x8 inch baking dish with olive oil. Pour in the batter. Bake at 325 degrees Fahrenheit for about 35 minutes, till a toothpick comes out clean.

Serves 16 portions

Banana & Blueberry Bread

3 mashed bananas

1 cup of blueberries

1 teaspoon of baking soda

1 teaspoon of baking powder

1 teaspoon of cinnamon

3 cups of almond flour

2 tablespoons of coconut flour

2 tablespoons of ground flaxseeds

½ teaspoon of salt

¼ cup of coconut milk

2 tablespoons of honey

1 tablespoon of vanilla extract

3 eggs

Coconut or olive oil for greasing

Prepare oven and heat it at 375 degrees Fahrenheit. Add coconut flour, almond flour, baking powder, baking soda, flaxseeds, salt and cinnamon in a large bowl. Whisk to combine.

Stir to mix the wet mixture with dry ingredients. Pour the final mixture into a greased loaf pan. Bake in the oven for 45 to 50 minutes.

Remove from the oven. Let it cool. Slice and serve in a plate.

Serves 1 loaf

Blackberry Bars

1 cup of coconut flour

½ cup of shredded coconut

1 teaspoon of cinnamon

½ teaspoon of baking soda

1 teaspoon of baking powder

½ teaspoon of sea salt

¼ cup of honey

2 bananas

2 eggs

2 tablespoons of melted coconut oil

1 teaspoon of vanilla extract

1 cup of almond milk

1 cup of fresh or frozen blackberries or any other berries

Prepare oven and heat it at 350 degrees Fahrenheit. Grease an 8x8 inch sized baking pan.

Mix shredded coconut, coconut flour, cinnamon, salt, baking soda and baking powder in a large bowl. Add honey and mix again. Add in eggs, bananas, vanilla extract, ¼ cup of the almond milk and coconut oil. Mix thoroughly. Add more almond milk if needed. The goal is to get a good consistency for the batter.

Fold in the berries. Spoon the batter into greased pan. Bake 40 minutes till they turn golden.

Remove from the oven. Cool. Cut into 16 squares.

Serves 16 squares

Blueberry Banana Boats

2 Bananas, unpeeled

½ cup of blueberries

½ cup of chopped walnuts

½ cup of shredded coconut

2 tablespoons of honey

Preheat the oven to 400 degrees Fahrenheit. Cut bananas open lengthwise while making sure not to cut through the peel on the other side. Stuff the blueberries into the bananas. Wrap them with aluminum foil. Seal at the top so they'll be easy to open.

 Place the bananas into the oven to cook for 10 minutes. Remove from the oven. Open up the tin foils and drizzle with honey. Serve.

Serves 2

Carrot Cookies

1 cup of chopped carrots

1 cup of almonds

½ cup of shredded coconut

½ teaspoon of nutmeg

1 teaspoon of vanilla extract

1 teaspoon of coconut oil

2 Eggs

Preheat the oven to 350 degrees Fahrenheit. Combine all ingredients in a food processor, except the eggs. Pulse till you end up with small pieces. Combine this mixture with eggs in a large bowl. Mix well. Form it into cookie shape with your hands. Place them on a cookie sheet lined with parchment paper.

Bake for 35 to 40 minutes till done.

Serves about 12 small cookies